A Cancer Battle Plan

Hope In A Fight You Didn't Pick

Joan L. Exline, PhD

ISBN-13: 978-1490511894
ISBN-10: 149051189Xd

Dedication

This book is dedicated to my family. Thank you for the prayers and unselfish support you gave me. You were my strength and encouragement when I needed it most.

Contents

Introduction   i

The Dreaded Words   1

Making My Choice   3

Selecting Your Medical Team   11

Where Else Is It?   13

Getting Ready   18

Starting Treatment   27

Living During Treatment   31

One Year Anniversary   38

From Joan's Husband and Family   40

About the Author   44

Introduction

Just Four Words

Written by Steve Green, Joan's husband

How many words do you think you speak in a day? How many words are spoken to you in a day? Most often in the course of a day, words are used to express ideas or convey thoughts or feelings about something or someone. Someone's reaction or response to words is governed by time, place, person, and situation.

In the pages and chapters ahead, you will experience the effects of words on someone's life. Joan Exline was a remarkable woman. She was a consummate professional, wife, sister, aunt, friend, and mentor who went about her daily activities with determination and purpose to improve anything she encountered. She was extremely adroit at assessing a situation or events around her and then working to improve them. She did not do this with the intent of personal recognition but instead as her way of making a contribution.

Joan was well respected by her peers, friends, and family. Her indomitable spirit and zest for life positively altered educational institutions, aided businesses to be more efficient, and profoundly affected the people she met along the way.

Early one evening in late July 2011, Joan received a phone call. Her (our) world would be inextricably changed by twelve letters. The twelve letters formed four simple words. The words she heard and relayed to me were:

You have a mass

What follows is Joan's journey in the aftermath of those four words.

The Dreaded Words

You can't believe it. The words you never thought you'd hear have been spoken. Yet, they <u>have</u> been spoken...and to you. That's right, this time it isn't about a friend, a colleague or a relative. It is about you. YOU HAVE CANCER!

And from this day on, your life will never be the same.

You don't know what to expect. You may be shocked and devastated. You are probably overwhelmed. You definitely are scared. No, not scared, you are terrified of the journey ahead of you.

But, how you respond ultimately is your decision. You may not realize it at first, but you are in charge of managing your journey. Yet, to truly take charge, you must learn as much as you can from the right sources and make good decisions.

Your journey begins with making the most important decision of all—how will you react? Yes, it IS a choice! You will need to make that choice over and over as new challenges confront you.

Sure, you can give up and stick your head in the sand. Or you can visualize the gloom and doom that might lie ahead. Or you can decide to fight, to be a warrior. It is your choice.

The purpose of this book is to identify some of the emotions and issues that face those diagnosed with cancer. It is not a substitute for medical care or treatment plans. Rather, it shares the experiences and emotions after I was diagnosed with pancreatic cancer and emphasizes the conversations that should take place with your physicians, family and friends.

Making My Choice

I first learned I had pancreatic cancer in July 2011, but the symptoms were there months earlier, just undetected. Two months before I began experiencing a dull abdominal pain after eating. We were on vacation at the time, and I thought maybe I had eaten too much rich food or drank too much wine. When things weren't better after we returned home to our normal routine and eating patterns, I went to see the doctor. My internist ordered the typical tests and procedures, ruling out one disease after another. Finally, the abdominal CT scan clearly identified a tumor on and nearby the pancreas. Further biopsies confirmed the tumor was malignant. I had pancreatic cancer.

I knew a little about pancreatic cancer and the poor odds of survival from stories in the media about Patrick Swayze and Steve Jobs. But, I needed to know more and began searching the internet. It didn't take long to confirm the bad news. Today, when we want and need information, we turn to the internet. There is no shortage of information there, and we can get to it 24 hours a day, 7 days a week. While the internet can help you understand your disease and develop a list of questions to discuss with your doctor, it also contains misleading information. Thus, it is very important to search with care and avoid self-diagnosis. I suggest starting with the National Cancer Institute site at www.cancer.gov.

One of the first pieces of information I frantically sought on the internet was data on survival rates. That's the first question most cancer victims ask. Am I going to live? How long?

Survival rates typically are based on a five-year period and are reported as the percentage of people with a given diagnosis that are still alive in five years. Likewise, the impact of treatment options are reported by identifying the number of months or years the treatment is likely to increase survival time. The survival rates for pancreatic cancer are dismal. Only a small percentage of the people diagnosed with pancreatic cancer live five years or longer. In part, this is because it is very difficult to diagnose pancreatic cancer so the disease is often well-advanced before treatment can be considered. In other words, cancerous tumors were likely growing inside my body well before my symptoms were detected in May 2011.

As you read about treatment options, you will also stumble upon the term *clinical trials,* and you may even be asked to participate in one. Clinical trials are scientific studies with rigorous guidelines that test how well treatment and medicines work in people. Many of the advances we have made in medicine are a result of clinical trials. You should carefully study and ask many questions about treatment options that have not been tested through clinical trials.

Clinical trials are divided into phases. Phase I trials test the best way to give a treatment and the proper dose. Phase II trials focus on the impact the treatment has on the disease. Phase III trials compare the results of those taking the treatment with those taking a standard treatment by randomly assigning people to receive the treatment or a placebo. Phase IV trials are undertaken to check for additional side effects across large numbers of people. (NCI Dictionary of Cancer Terms, 2012)

So when I searched for the survival rates and treatment options for pancreatic cancer, my head was swirling with data and clinical terms. Nothing looked promising. After hours of searching, I remember turning off my computer, deciding that none of this was for me. I was not going to fight this monster called pancreatic cancer when the odds of survival were so poor. I convinced myself that I was all about dying with dignity and began sharing my plans to die *my way* with family, friends and my doctors.

The doctors seemed surprised that I would give up. After all, I was only 54, in otherwise good health, with a promising career. Most importantly, I had recently married a great guy who very much wanted me alive and well, and I wanted to be alive and well with him. What they didn't know initially is that I had watched my late husband die from lung cancer in the year 2000. He went from a smart, vibrant, loving man to a paralyzed, uncommunicative vegetable as the cancer spread from his lungs to his spine to his brain. As his caregiver, my life was put on hold to deal with the horrors before us. There was one difference between us--he had the benefit of numbing pain medicine until he died while I watched his death unfold in high density detail.

I didn't want that type of death and long ago had made the decision that I would do nothing beyond reason to extend my life. I also didn't want to put my new husband, Steve, through the nightmare of dealing with my death.

Thus, I made my choice—instead of taking control of the cancer, I decided to let the cancer control me. In doing so, I decided to be a victim.

My husband didn't like this decision at all. We had only been married two years when I was diagnosed with cancer. Our life together was just beginning! On one hand, he wanted me to fight. On the other hand, he didn't want me to face pain and suffering by pursuing treatments I did not really want. He was torn by his desire for me to live versus wanting to be supportive of my wishes. We had no children together, so that wasn't a consideration for us but it would be for many cancer patients.

Fortunately, one of my physicians got through to me. He drilled into me that the poor odds of surviving pancreatic cancer didn't have to apply to me. The articles I had been reading were statistical studies; yet, I am not just a number, I am a person.

He said to me rather sternly, "You don't have to be that statistic. There have been survivors of every type of cancer." I thought about that. He made sense. Why can't I be a survivor?

He also explained to me that if I don't try the treatment options, I will never know if a given treatment works for me. Further, he convinced me that if I chose to try the treatment and didn't like the way it made me feel, I could always stop it. "You are in control", he insisted. I liked the sound of that.

Another physician guided my reading about pancreatic cancer to focus on more balanced articles so I could see there was hope amongst the challenges.

Then I began hearing from friends as the word of my diagnosis spread. One person told me about her battle with a rare form of ovarian cancer. According to the statistics, she was supposed to be dead years ago. Likewise, another person shared with me how her father was still alive and doing well after being diagnosed with Stage IV lung cancer *seven* years ago.

Those two physicians and stories from friends changed my way of thinking and altered my response to cancer. I began to have hope. With more time to think and pray, I revised my choice. It was then that I picked up my sword and chose to be a warrior rather than a victim.

Selecting Your Medical Team

Another important decision is where to go for care. I was fortunate to have access to a university research center, the University of South Alabama Mitchell Cancer Institute. While there are many quality cancer programs across the country, I personally believe it is important to pursue care (or at least get a consultation from) an institution that is also involved in research and has the latest equipment.

Likewise, it is important that you are comfortable with your physicians and medical providers. The ideal situation is to seek care at an institution that uses a team approach whereby a team of physicians is working on your behalf. The number and type of doctors involved in treating your cancer will depend on the type of cancer and resources available to you in your community. In my case, at least 4-6 physicians discussed my case regularly at their weekly team conferences.

The medical oncologist on your team is imperative. The medical oncologist often is the doctor that coordinates your care and manages the chemotherapy, if that's part of your treatment plan. It is very important that you can comfortably talk to your medical oncologist and that you are on the same page regarding issues like pain control and quality of life. If surgery is possible, your team may include a surgical oncologist. If radiation treatment is considered, a radiation oncologist will be on the team.

Other providers may include pediatric specialists (for children), pathologists and the clinical lab, oncology nurses and physician assistants. Additional support may be available from oncology social workers, rehabilitation therapists, dietitians, psychiatrists, pharmacists and chaplains.

Where Else Is It?

Before we could prepare my treatment (battle) plan, it was important to know where else the cancer might be in my body. This was determined by having a Positron Emission Tomography (PET) scan. The PET scan is an imaging technique that produces a three-dimensional image or picture of functional processes in the body. In modern scanners, three dimensional imaging is often accomplished with the aid of a Commuted Tomography (CT) scan performed during the same session, in the same machine. Together, the scan helps to identify tumors and possible cancer metastasis (spreading).

I had my first PET scan in August 2011. The preparation for the PET scan involved very specific dietary restrictions the day and night before. The next morning, the staff inserted intravenous material and had me wait in a dark, quiet room while the contrast material circulated throughout my body. After about an hour, it was time for the scan. I found it very helpful to record relaxation music on my iPod before the scan. Once in the quiet room, listening to the music helped me relax and pass the time. Since I'm terribly claustrophobic, the calming music was also helpful (along with sedation) during the actual scan.

Then it was time for more "waiting." You might as well accept up front that waiting is a big part of cancer and cancer treatment. It helps if you have a team of family and friends that can alternate their support and waiting time with you. I was lucky to have my husband and a number of supportive friends. For the big tests, my younger sister in Indianapolis always flew in to be with me. That meant a lot. No matter how strong you think you are, you need someone by your side to worry with you, laugh with you and cope with the fear. You also may need help with transportation.

That night, the preliminary PET report gave us the news that spawned both hope and grief within me. The good news was that the cancer was localized to the area surrounding the pancreas. The bad news--the grief-- was that the cancer was too big amidst all those tiny arteries and veins for surgery. With many types of cancer, surgery will be done right away to remove the tumor, followed by chemotherapy and possibly radiation. Pancreatic cancer is different when the cancer has grown outside the pancreas, making surgery too risky.

Finding middle ground, I was told it was possible that chemotherapy and/or radiation could shrink the tumor to the point where surgery might be possible. At minimum, the chemo and radiation could reduce the size of the tumor (thereby reducing my pain) and prevent it from spreading. It was time to make another choice. I chose to focus on the hope of chemotherapy and radiation rather than the grief of not being eligible for surgery.

Given the PET results, the next step was to get the port installed in my chest to make it easier to administer chemotherapy. As I was prepped in outpatient surgery, it hit me. This is really happening. I have cancer and now I need a port for chemotherapy. Prior to surgery, I found myself watching other people do normal things and thinking, *"How can they go to the store or talk calmly on their cell phone as they drive down the street? Don't they know I have CANCER?"* The outpatient surgery team at USA Medical Center seemed to understand that. They worked hard to make me comfortable, and the nurse anesthetist even got me to laugh.

As I woke up in recovery and prepared to leave, the recovery nurse stopped what she was doing and looked me in the eye. She said, "You have a journey ahead of you. Prepare for the worst but then forget that and focus on the positive. You have to think positively." She planted a seed of hope in me, and I never forgot her words.

The next day, my husband accompanied me to see the medical oncologist. We left his office with a plan -- at last, a battle plan! The treatment protocol chosen by my physicians during their team conference involved 17 weeks that included four chemotherapy treatments two weeks apart, a three week break, then 10 days of radiation therapy coupled with weekly chemotherapy. Although I was scared beyond words, actually having a battle plan brought me comfort.

Getting Ready

When I learned chemotherapy was part of my battle plan, I had two thoughts: (1) I'd vomit all the time and (2) I'd lose my hair. In fact, about 30% of the people getting my "chemo cocktail" lose their hair or experience some thinning. I have very thick hair, so my husband jokingly commented, "Well, you pay to have your hair cut every three weeks now, so that savings should make you happy!" I didn't laugh. Some things just aren't funny when you have cancer.

During the educational session prior to starting chemotherapy, the nurse told me that how people react to chemotherapy varies. She said that she has observed two people with the same type and stage of cancer get the same treatment and respond in two different ways. She suggested it was all about being hardy. The patients who were hardy and approached treatment with a positive attitude tended to do better. Of course, some chemicals are so harsh that side effects are impossible to avoid. But, her words made me reach within and shore up my internal hardiness.

My hair dresser, Elaine, who is also a good friend, went on alert. First, we went wig shopping in the catalogs to look for a fun hair style that I could never have managed with my natural hair. She said that if we began to see hair loss on the horizon, we'd clip my natural hair during the transition and then move into a wig as it started to fall out. Again, I had another plan that minimized my worries!

My younger sister challenged the rest of the females in my family to shave their heads in support. I didn't want that! I protested! Fortunately, the others also convinced her that this wasn't a good idea. I will fast-forward and tell you that I didn't lose my hair at all. However, I was ready and that made me feel good... and the females in my family were very happy they didn't listen to my sister! Can you imagine if they had shaved their heads and then I didn't lose my hair?

I also learned that there are many medications out there for nausea. If taken properly, there is little need to fear nausea. The oncology nurses are trained to work with you on what to eat and how to use these wonderful medications to reduce struggles with vomiting and diarrhea.

Thus, chemotherapy isn't always as bad as it used to be.

Like it or not, it is important to consider the worst case - that you will die. You should have an Advanced Directive that reflects your wishes and is properly prepared to meet your state's requirements. Otherwise, your family and medical team will likely do everything possible to save you in an emergency situation. In other words, you need to think about your wishes, discuss them with your family and appropriately document them. Likewise, it is important that the Advanced Directive be readily accessible if it is needed. Some Advanced Directives may be too general, and you will want to consider making a detailed list of procedures that you don't want, such as defibrillation, rather than just talking generally about life saving measures.

It doesn't do you any good for this document to be locked away in a bank safe if you need it on a weekend. Because my husband and I married later in life, many of our financial affairs remain separate. To make things easier for him, I put all important documents--my Will, records of my accounts, etc.--in one drawer so they would be easily accessible to him.

It also is important to confront your death. For some, this is a time of fear. For others, it is important to understand the dying process and the pain that may go with it. If you fall in the latter category, this is a good time to learn about hospice services and get reassurance that many things can be done to make your death peaceful and painless. You also need to decide about funeral services, burial or cremation preferences, and other end of life decisions.

I chose to confront my death by thinking not only about the pragmatic decisions that had to be made but also about life decisions I had made over the years. Had I been a good person? Had I made a difference to others? More importantly, did I tell others they made a difference to me? There definitely were words I wanted to share with those I loved. This approach sometimes made people uncomfortable because they wanted me to focus on living rather than dying. In that case, to avoid discomfort, you can leave written notes for those you love to open after your death. My late husband did that for me, and it meant a lot for me to know when I was deep in mourning that he wanted me to go on with my life and be happy again.

My younger sister seemed to understand this need to assess the value of my life and came up with a great Christmas present for me. She made a VoiceQuilt by asking people in my past and present life to call in and record a memory. She enlisted the help of friends during various phases of my life to come up with a good representation over my 54 years! My eyes were filled with tears as I listened to my VoiceQuilt on Christmas day and realized how many "good memories" I had made over the years. I felt I had touched the lives of others in a valuable way. (To learn more about VoiceQuilt, visit www.voicequilt.com.)

As I read about death and dying, it became clear that the battle with cancer included positive thinking. I read several books that cited evidence of beating diseases like cancer with positive thinking. There were accounts of people living that should have died and people dying that might have lived. In fact, after reading these stories, there were times that I was afraid that I was not thinking positively enough and that might hasten my death. This provoked much anxiety within me. Finally, one of my physicians assured me that having an occasional negative thought was normal and would not cause me to die faster.

No matter how hard I focused on positive thinking and hope, however, I struggled with why I was stricken with cancer. I believe in God and that there is a better place for me. I also was at peace with what happens after I die, but I feared the actual act of dying. I don't want to lie in bed and gasp for air as my lungs fill with fluid. I don't want to be unconscious and have people hovering over me, stroking my hand. I don't want to be hot or hurt and not be able to express my needs for relief. Most of all, I don't want to lose my mind and be a vegetable.

I talked with my minister about this struggle. Pastor Jeff listened carefully and then calmly told me, "It sounds like you have the after-life part all figured out so you don't need to think about that anymore. You can let people know how you feel about the act of dying right now while you are able to express yourself." He continued, "So have those conversations and file that "peace with dying" feeling away. Begin to focus your energy, thoughts and prayers on getting well." Pastor Jeff is pretty good about simple but profound advice like that.

At Pastor Jeff's suggestion, I also read a book titled "Making Sense of God's Will" by Adam Hamilton. I recommend it. Not everyone believes the same things but I've come to the conclusion that (1) I don't have cancer for a predetermined reason and (2) I haven't done anything to deserve cancer or the suffering associated with it. Yes, I have made mistakes, but I have asked for and believe I have received forgiveness for my sins. Therefore, I am not destined to have cancer and since it isn't my destiny, I should fight it. I can also be at peace because I know that God will be with me along the way and will lead me to a far better life when I leave this life.

That's what I believe. Your beliefs may be different. Regardless, I encourage you to figure out what you believe, to find your faith and rely on it to get you through the tough times ahead. The experience of that alone will change you.

Starting Treatment

It is a very strange feeling when you first sit in the chemo chair and realize they are pumping poisonous chemicals in you. One of my dear friends who is also a cancer survivor helped me deal with that. She told me to think of the chemo as Pac Man, the fun creature from the electronic games of the 70s and 80s, chomping away on my cancer cells. It was perfect imagery that helped me think positively during my chemo sessions! In fact, there were moments during the weeks when I didn't have chemo that I worried about not having Pac Man at work within me.

By this time, my whole world was filtered through the eyes of cancer. It is odd how when you have cancer you start looking at things in a different way. Not only do you need time to adjust, but your friends, family and colleagues need time to get over the shock, too.

My schedule became dictated by appointments for procedures and treatments. All I could think about was cancer. In fact, I sometimes got disturbed when someone talked to me about something ordinary. How can they think about ordinary matters when I have cancer? I found that I needed a quiet place where I could absorb all that was happening to me and where I could pray to God and gather strength. There were other times when I wanted people to quit asking me questions, especially when I didn't know the answers. All I can say is that you just need to tell people when you do and don't want to talk about it.

I also needed the support of my friends, but I quickly learned that I didn't have the energy to tell my story over and over again. Thus, I created a Caring Bridge account at www.caringbridge.org so I could keep my friends and family informed. Little did I know that I would get so much in return from all the posts in my guestbook --- advice, shared memories from other cancer survivors, good jokes to take my mind off of cancer and many, many words of inspiration.

I also began to look for signs. My mom died of dementia-related complications in October 2009. She loved yellow roses. Whether my dad had money for one rose or a dozen roses, he would present her with yellow roses on special occasions. The day after I was told I had a mass of some sort in my pancreatic area, my emotions were raw. But, I tried to do normal things and went to a local grocery store to pick up a few things. It was Saturday, the day when various kids' groups "bag for donations." That particular Saturday, the young teenagers were raising money for their World Series baseball trip to the state of Washington.

I put three dollars in their collection bucket, and one of the kids went to a basket full of long stem roses. Puzzled, I watched him as he first selected a pink rose, put it back, then selected a yellow rose and presented it to me for my donation. Needless to say, I thought of my mom watching over me and the tears began to flow. When he grows up, that poor kid will probably never buy his future girlfriend or wife roses without thinking of that crazy lady at the grocery store! However, the story doesn't end there. The next weekend, as my husband was reading the sports scores in the newspaper, he shouted for me to join him in the living room. Amazingly, the local team won the World Series! As you can imagine, I took it as a sign and shed many tears that morning.

Being alert to signs is okay. It fosters hope. Even the strongest of warriors need signs of hope!

Living During Treatment

This sounds simple, but it is hard to do -- you need to keep living during your treatment.

When I found out that surgery wasn't an option, I went to Plan B, which was chemotherapy, followed by a few weeks of radiation and then many, many more chemotherapy treatments. During this time, I had to learn to live with the effects of the cancer itself and the treatment.

Keeping Busy

For me, living during treatment meant continuing to work and being a wife. While it was difficult to arrange treatments around my work schedule, it could be done. I worked all day and had chemo and radiation at the end of the day. I scheduled the chemo treatments for Fridays so I could have the weekend to partially recover. For me, going to work every day gave me purpose. When things were really bad, I knew I could take vacation or sick time. But, for most days, I needed the distraction of going to work.

As for my role as a wife, I also tried to do things that my husband liked to do. Before I was sick, we loved to play golf every weekend, take trips to the beach, go out to eat regularly, walk our three poodles and go to church on Sundays. Cancer not only affects you, it affects your spouse and family. Just as with me, suddenly Steve's life changed dramatically. I tried to do our normal activities as much as I could, but that isn't easy and sometimes impossible. Chemotherapy made it difficult for me to enjoy eating and I eventually had to quit playing golf for a while. However, I did what I could and I encouraged my husband to play golf with others and have time away from "cancer and sickness."

Pain

Pain was a real problem. Hopefully, if you are fighting cancer, pain won't be a major part of your disease. But, for many types of cancer, especially pancreatic cancer, pain is an ongoing nightmare. Once again, there are many options out there to reduce your pain - pills, Opium patches, nerve injections, and narcotic pumps to name a few. Pain treatments can make you sleepy and can cause serious side effects such as constipation, so talk to your doctor about options that will allow you to continue to be comfortable as long as you can. In some cases, you may need to see a pain specialist. As one of my friends who survived cancer told me, there is no reason to be in pain from cancer in this day and age. There are options! If one doesn't work, be aggressive in seeking additional or alternative options. If your doctor won't listen to you, find one who will.

Emotions

Cancer and the pain that you face challenges your emotions as you undertake your journey. I was a person who seldom cried, yet dealing with cancer made me cry when I least expected it. If you find yourself in this situation, don't hesitate to seek help. It is normal to need help. Ask your doctor for a referral to a psychiatrist who hopefully can also be part of your cancer team.

Holidays can be particularly challenging for your emotions. For example, you may be worried that this will be your last holiday with family members, but then you find out that they have other things they want to do. They may want to take a vacation or feel they need to spend time with in-laws. It makes sense but it still hurts. You'll need someone to talk through these types of situations with you.

Another emotional issue is your family and spouse. I had to learn that people couldn't read my mind. They didn't know that when I responded that I was "okay" I was sometimes really saying I needed their help. My husband's best friend was talking about this with me one day and advised me that I had to find a way to express what I really needed my husband to do. That isn't always easy. I'd rather he could sense my every need. But, sometimes, I just had to tell him. Again, sometimes you'll need a professional to talk about this type of thing with you and maybe even your spouse or family.

Visitors

My family and friends are scattered across the country so getting together in person wasn't easy to do. I was fortunate to have friends in Mobile, and later my older sister moved to Mobile. For those that lived far away, I was touched that many family and friends wanted to come be with me through the treatment, and others wanted to come during special times for inspiration and encouragement. I've been very lucky to have this support.

The problem is that visitors don't always realize that their visit needs to be different from the normal get-togethers when you were healthy and simply entertaining. You are undergoing treatments and trying to "live", both of which drain you of the strength to get through the day, much less the energy needed to entertain guests. Likewise, your spouse and other caregivers may be worn out. Somehow, you need to communicate to out of town friends and family that you'd love them to be with you, but they have to come as helpers, not as guests. If you have difficulty communicating this, delegate it to a family member or friend that can intervene for you. My younger sister took on this role for me and Steve.

Support and Encouragement

I mentioned using CaringBridge (www.caringbridge.org) as a means to communicate with family and friends. I can't tell you how valuable it has been to read words of support throughout my journey. One friend from long ago in high school in Indiana, Denise, would send me cards that always managed to arrive on chemo days and big decision days (days when I had a scan to check my status).

Besides messages of encouragement, people would write to me about how I had influenced their lives and how my approach to dealing with pancreatic cancer was inspiring them in their own lives. These words of support and encouragement made me feel that my battle with cancer mattered and spurred me on. I can never thank enough all those people who wrote to me via the CaringBridge guestbook, Facebook, text messages and regular email. Although I tried, I know I couldn't answer them all. But, they all meant so very much to me.

One Year Anniversary

It is May 2012, and one year since I first felt the pain that went undetected for another two months. Once the diagnosis of Stage 3 pancreatic cancer was made, I underwent a protocol of chemotherapy and radiation over the next 5 months. After a promising CT scan in December 2011, I took 4 weeks off. My next PET scan was done on February 6, 2012. The PET scan showed the disease had not spread and the tumor showed less metabolic activity. Both results were very good signs that I was winning the battle. From mid-January through mid-May, I continued with biweekly Gemcitabine (marketed as Gemzar) chemotherapy. The doctors preferred that I take chemo every 3 of 4 weeks during this phase, but my counts would fall and my quality of life was not good. We compromised and agreed to every other week.

May 9, 2012 is the next PET scan. I've decided that there will be choices to make, depending on the results.

<ADD RESULTS AND CHOICE>

(This was Joan's placeholder and last entry)

From Joan's Family

The PET scan on May 9th didn't show positive results. The pancreatic cancer tumor had increased in both size and density. We spent a long time discussing three options with her physicians:

Option 1—do nothing. The tumor would spread first to her liver, and then it would be rampant throughout her body. Joan talks in this book about "how long do I have to live." The results from this PET scan couldn't be classified. Her death could occur in weeks or months.

Option 2—a Level 2 chemo defense. This would be a much harsher chemo regiment that had high likelihood of negative side effects— sores on her fingers and toes to the point where she couldn't work on her computer, etc. Being able to continue to work and contribute at the University of South Alabama gave her strength throughout her battle, so going with this route of chemo took her driving force away from her. As with her Level 1 chemo defense, at some point her tumor would become resistant to the Level 2 chemo cocktail, so all in all she eliminated this option.

Option 3—a clinical trial. At first, there weren't any trial matches that fit Joan's particular stage and type of pancreatic cancer. Then, her wonderful radiation oncologist, Dr. Suzanne Russo, found a clinical trial at John Hopkins in Baltimore, MD, that fit Joan perfectly.

Joan was excited at first about furthering pancreatic cancer research by participating in a clinical trial, but soon her extreme claustrophobia and anxiety spun out of control. By late June 2012, she could only be a passenger in a car if all four windows were rolled down and the driver stopped the car every 5 minutes to let her get out of the car for a bit.

Her anxiety was such that she had to keep moving, every second of every moment awake. It was exhausting for her loved ones around her, and Joan often didn't sleep more than minutes at time.

Joan's pain was so constant and intense that she couldn't eat more than five bites of food a day over several days. By early July, it became impossible to consider any potential logistics to get Joan from Mobile, AL to Baltimore, MD for the clinical trial.

We unfortunately lost Joan on July 26, 2012, and as painful as it is for us to be here without her, we are comforted to know she is now pain free and at peace.

Joan mentions in this book the importance of being at a facility that not only provides care but also is involved in research. In late 2011, Joan established the Exline Pancreatic Cancer Scientific Investigation Fund in conjunction with the University of South Alabama and the USA Mitchell Cancer Institute. All proceeds from this book will be given to the fund that Joan established.

If you would like to make additional contributions to this fund, such contributions may be made to the Exline Pancreatic Cancer Scientific Investigation Fund, University of South Alabama Development Office, 650 Clinic Drive, Mobile, AL, 36688-0002.

Her family extends a heartfelt thank you to the Infusion Staff at USA Mitchell Cancer Center and Drs. Butler, Russo, and Contreras for the excellent care and attention that was provided to Joan.

About the Author

Joan L. Exline, Ph.D. passed away on July 26th after a hard fought battle with pancreatic cancer. Joan was born on February 13, 1957 as the third of four children to the late M. Joan Exline and Eugene V. Exline in Evansville, IN. She grew up in Evansville, IN, graduating from F.J. Reitz High School in 1975. She went on to earn a B. S. in Business from Indiana University and a master's degree in health administration from the University of Michigan. After working as a hospital administrator in the Midwest for a number of years, she returned to Wayne State University to earn a doctorate in public policy, specializing in health policy. In 1997, she completed a fellowship in health services research with Duke University and the Department of Veteran Affairs.

In addition to being the Principal Consultant of J Exline & Associates consulting firm, serving on several healthcare, educational, and professional publications' committees and boards, and teaching health policy and administration at several universities, Joan held several positions during her successful eleven year career at the University of Southern Mississippi, including Graduate Program Director; Director, Department of Community Health Sciences; Interim Dean, College of Health; and Assistant to the President— Accreditation, Planning, and Articulation.

Joan moved to Mobile, AL, to join the University of South Alabama in 2008 as AVP of Institutional Research, Planning, Assessment and Regional Campuses while also teaching online graduate health administration and policy courses within the MPA program. She was instrumental in revamping processes and practices to bring the University into compliance with SACS Principles and directed all necessary requirements to achieve SACS accreditation. While there, she also chaired numerous committees and developed new programs within the University.

Joan was honored numerous times during her storied career, including the Mississippi Institutions of Higher Learning Best Practices Award, Strong Woman of Mississippi— Leadership, and CHHS Distinguished Teaching Award. She authored several professional publications and articles.

Joan was a member of Christ United Methodist Church in Mobile, AL and various professional organizations.

CPSIA information can be obtained at www.ICGtesting.com
Printed in the USA
LVOW08s2135040914

402553LV00013B/167/P